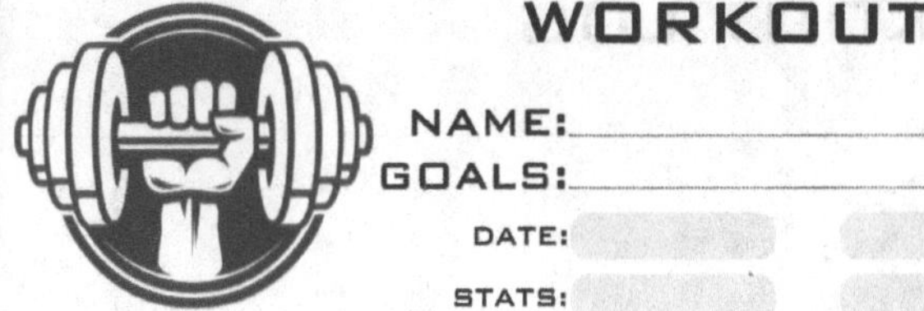

WORKOUT LOG

NAME:
GOALS:
DATE:
STATS:
WEIGHT:

EXERCISE:	SETS	REPS	WEIGHT	REST	SETS	REPS	WEIGHT	REST	SETS	REPS	WEIGHT	REST	SETS	REPS	WEIGHT	REST

CARDIO:	TIME	DIST.	INT.	PACE	TIME	DIST.	INT.	PACE	TIME	DIST.	INT.	PACE	TIME	DIST.	INT.	PACE

WORKOUT LOG

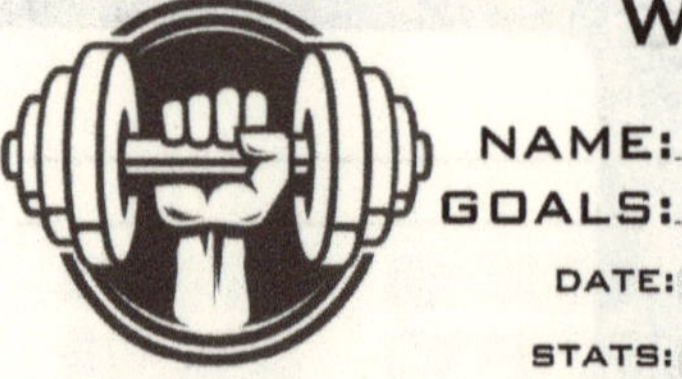

NAME:

GOALS:

DATE:

STATS:

WEIGHT:

EXERCISE:	SETS	REPS	WEIGHT	REST	SETS	REPS	WEIGHT	REST	SETS	REPS	WEIGHT	REST	SETS	REPS	WEIGHT	REST

CARDIO:	TIME	DIST.	INT.	PACE	TIME	DIST.	INT.	PACE	TIME	DIST.	INT.	PACE	TIME	DIST.	INT.	PACE

WORKOUT LOG

NAME:

GOALS:

DATE:

STATS:

WEIGHT:

EXERCISE:	SETS	REPS	WEIGHT	REST	SETS	REPS	WEIGHT	REST	SETS	REPS	WEIGHT	REST	SETS	REPS	WEIGHT	REST

CARDIO:	TIME	DIST.	INT.	PACE	TIME	DIST.	INT.	PACE	TIME	DIST.	INT.	PACE	TIME	DIST.	INT.	PACE

WORKOUT LOG

NAME:
GOALS:
DATE:
STATS:
WEIGHT:

EXERCISE:	SETS	REPS	WEIGHT	REST	SETS	REPS	WEIGHT	REST	SETS	REPS	WEIGHT	REST	SETS	REPS	WEIGHT	REST

CARDIO:	TIME	DIST.	INT.	PACE	TIME	DIST.	INT.	PACE	TIME	DIST.	INT.	PACE	TIME	DIST.	INT.	PACE

WORKOUT LOG

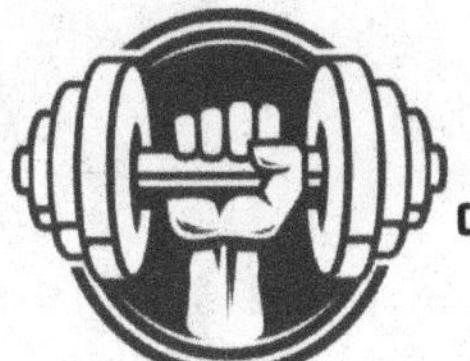

NAME:

GOALS:

DATE:

STATS:

WEIGHT:

EXERCISE:	SETS	REPS	WEIGHT	REST	SETS	REPS	WEIGHT	REST	SETS	REPS	WEIGHT	REST	SETS	REPS	WEIGHT	REST

CARDIO:	TIME	DIST.	INT.	PACE	TIME	DIST.	INT.	PACE	TIME	DIST.	INT.	PACE	TIME	DIST.	INT.	PACE

WORKOUT LOG

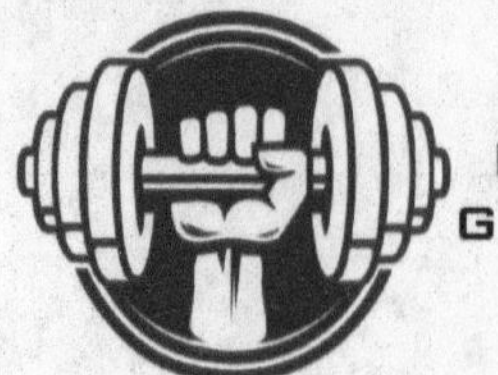

NAME:

GOALS:

DATE:

STATS:

WEIGHT:

EXERCISE:	SETS	REPS	WEIGHT	REST	SETS	REPS	WEIGHT	REST	SETS	REPS	WEIGHT	REST	SETS	REPS	WEIGHT	REST

CARDIO:	TIME	DIST.	INT.	PACE	TIME	DIST.	INT.	PACE	TIME	DIST.	INT.	PACE	TIME	DIST.	INT.	PACE

WORKOUT LOG

NAME:
GOALS:
DATE:
STATS:
WEIGHT:

EXERCISE:	SETS	REPS	WEIGHT	REST	SETS	REPS	WEIGHT	REST	SETS	REPS	WEIGHT	REST	SETS	REPS	WEIGHT	REST

CARDIO:	TIME	DIST.	INT.	PACE	TIME	DIST.	INT.	PACE	TIME	DIST.	INT.	PACE	TIME	DIST.	INT.	PACE

WORKOUT LOG

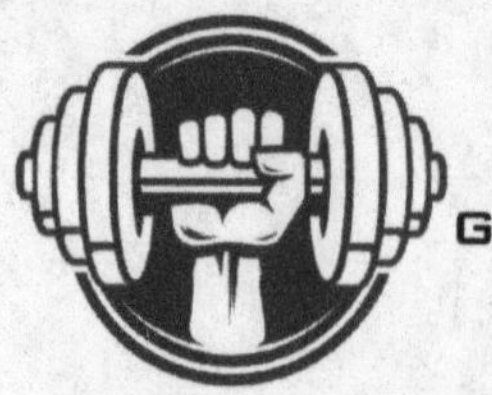

NAME:

GOALS:

DATE:

STATS:

WEIGHT:

EXERCISE:	SETS	REPS	WEIGHT	REST	SETS	REPS	WEIGHT	REST	SETS	REPS	WEIGHT	REST	SETS	REPS	WEIGHT	REST

CARDIO:	TIME	DIST.	INT.	PACE	TIME	DIST.	INT.	PACE	TIME	DIST.	INT.	PACE	TIME	DIST.	INT.	PACE

WORKOUT LOG

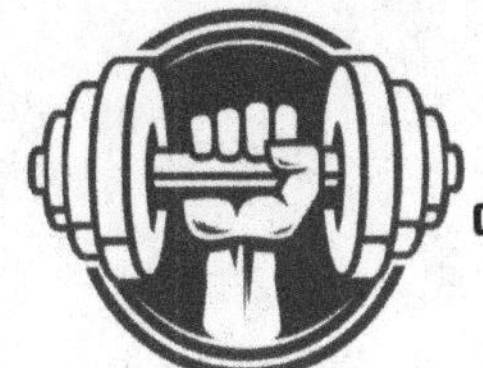

NAME:

GOALS:

DATE:

STATS:

WEIGHT:

EXERCISE:	SETS	REPS	WEIGHT	REST	SETS	REPS	WEIGHT	REST	SETS	REPS	WEIGHT	REST	SETS	REPS	WEIGHT	REST

CARDIO:	TIME	DIST.	INT.	PACE	TIME	DIST.	INT.	PACE	TIME	DIST.	INT.	PACE	TIME	DIST.	INT.	PACE

WORKOUT LOG

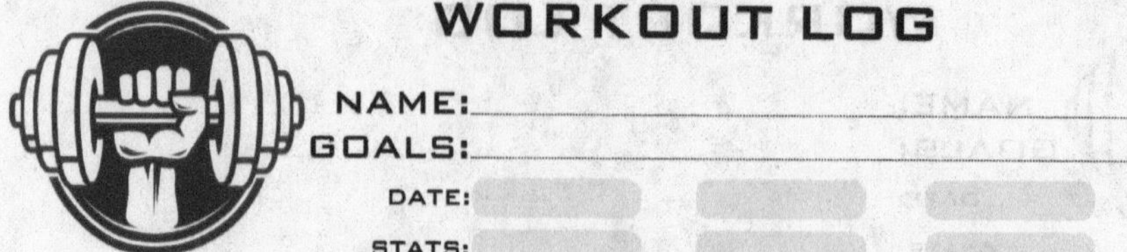

NAME:

GOALS:

DATE:

STATS:

WEIGHT:

EXERCISE:	SETS	REPS	WEIGHT	REST	SETS	REPS	WEIGHT	REST	SETS	REPS	WEIGHT	REST	SETS	REPS	WEIGHT	REST

CARDIO:	TIME	DIST.	INT.	PACE	TIME	DIST.	INT.	PACE	TIME	DIST.	INT.	PACE	TIME	DIST.	INT.	PACE

WORKOUT LOG

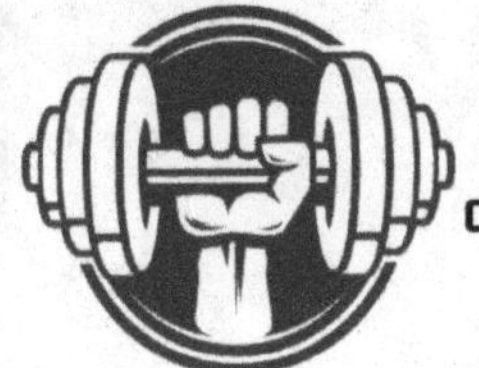

NAME:

GOALS:

DATE:

STATS:

WEIGHT:

EXERCISE:	SETS	REPS	WEIGHT	REST	SETS	REPS	WEIGHT	REST	SETS	REPS	WEIGHT	REST	SETS	REPS	WEIGHT	REST

CARDIO:	TIME	DIST.	INT.	PACE	TIME	DIST.	INT.	PACE	TIME	DIST.	INT.	PACE	TIME	DIST.	INT.	PACE

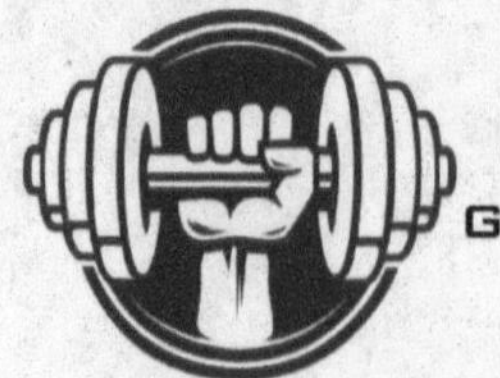

WORKOUT LOG

NAME:
GOALS:
DATE:
STATS:
WEIGHT:

EXERCISE:	SETS	REPS	WEIGHT	REST	SETS	REPS	WEIGHT	REST	SETS	REPS	WEIGHT	REST	SETS	REPS	WEIGHT	REST

CARDIO:	TIME	DIST.	INT.	PACE	TIME	DIST.	INT.	PACE	TIME	DIST.	INT.	PACE	TIME	DIST.	INT.	PACE

WORKOUT LOG

NAME:
GOALS:
DATE:
STATS:
WEIGHT:

EXERCISE:	SETS	REPS	WEIGHT	REST	SETS	REPS	WEIGHT	REST	SETS	REPS	WEIGHT	REST	SETS	REPS	WEIGHT	REST

CARDIO:	TIME	DIST.	INT.	PACE	TIME	DIST.	INT.	PACE	TIME	DIST.	INT.	PACE	TIME	DIST.	INT.	PACE

WORKOUT LOG

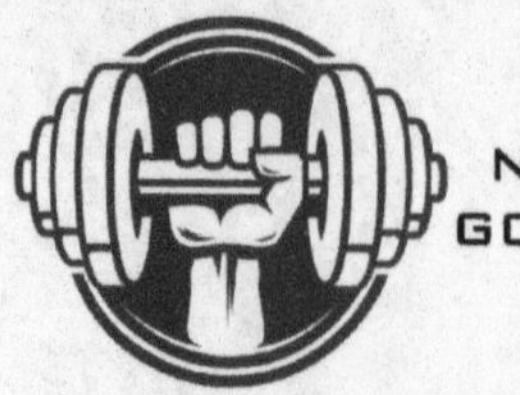

NAME:

GOALS:

DATE:

STATS:

WEIGHT:

EXERCISE:	SETS	REPS	WEIGHT	REST	SETS	REPS	WEIGHT	REST	SETS	REPS	WEIGHT	REST	SETS	REPS	WEIGHT	REST

CARDIO:	TIME	DIST.	INT.	PACE	TIME	DIST.	INT.	PACE	TIME	DIST.	INT.	PACE	TIME	DIST.	INT.	PACE

WORKOUT LOG

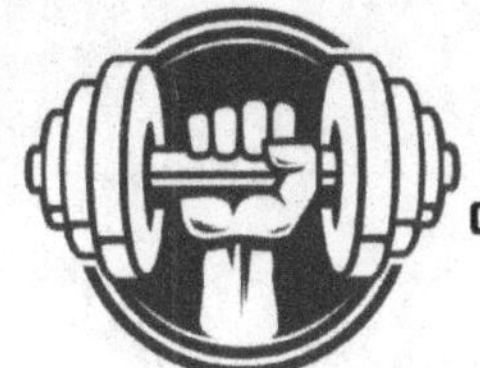

NAME:

GOALS:

DATE:

STATS:

WEIGHT:

EXERCISE:	SETS	REPS	WEIGHT	REST	SETS	REPS	WEIGHT	REST	SETS	REPS	WEIGHT	REST	SETS	REPS	WEIGHT	REST

CARDIO:	TIME	DIST.	INT.	PACE	TIME	DIST.	INT.	PACE	TIME	DIST.	INT.	PACE	TIME	DIST.	INT.	PACE

WORKOUT LOG

NAME: ______________________________

GOALS: ______________________________

DATE: ______________________________

STATS: ______________________________

WEIGHT: ______________________________

EXERCISE:	SETS	REPS	WEIGHT	REST	SETS	REPS	WEIGHT	REST	SETS	REPS	WEIGHT	REST	SETS	REPS	WEIGHT	REST

CARDIO:	TIME	DIST.	INT.	PACE	TIME	DIST.	INT.	PACE	TIME	DIST.	INT.	PACE	TIME	DIST.	INT.	PACE

WORKOUT LOG

NAME:

GOALS:

DATE:

STATS:

WEIGHT:

EXERCISE:	SETS	REPS	WEIGHT	REST	SETS	REPS	WEIGHT	REST	SETS	REPS	WEIGHT	REST	SETS	REPS	WEIGHT	REST

CARDIO:	TIME	DIST.	INT.	PACE	TIME	DIST.	INT.	PACE	TIME	DIST.	INT.	PACE	TIME	DIST.	INT.	PACE

WORKOUT LOG

NAME:

GOALS:

DATE:

STATS:

WEIGHT:

EXERCISE:	SETS	REPS	WEIGHT	REST	SETS	REPS	WEIGHT	REST	SETS	REPS	WEIGHT	REST	SETS	REPS	WEIGHT	REST

CARDIO:	TIME	DIST.	INT.	PACE	TIME	DIST.	INT.	PACE	TIME	DIST.	INT.	PACE	TIME	DIST.	INT.	PACE

WORKOUT LOG

NAME:
GOALS:
DATE:
STATS:
WEIGHT:

EXERCISE:	SETS	REPS	WEIGHT	REST	SETS	REPS	WEIGHT	REST	SETS	REPS	WEIGHT	REST	SETS	REPS	WEIGHT	REST

CARDIO:	TIME	DIST.	INT.	PACE	TIME	DIST.	INT.	PACE	TIME	DIST.	INT.	PACE	TIME	DIST.	INT.	PACE

WORKOUT LOG

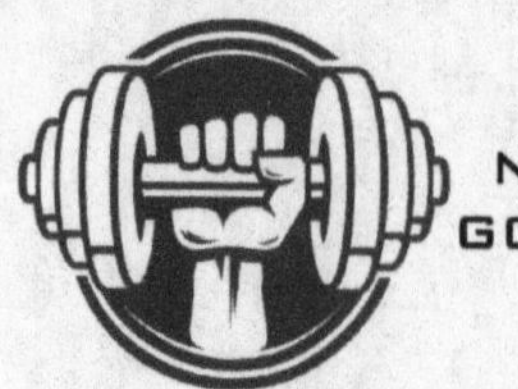

NAME:

GOALS:

DATE:

STATS:

WEIGHT:

EXERCISE:	SETS	REPS	WEIGHT	REST	SETS	REPS	WEIGHT	REST	SETS	REPS	WEIGHT	REST	SETS	REPS	WEIGHT	REST

CARDIO:	TIME	DIST.	INT.	PACE	TIME	DIST.	INT.	PACE	TIME	DIST.	INT.	PACE	TIME	DIST.	INT.	PACE

WORKOUT LOG

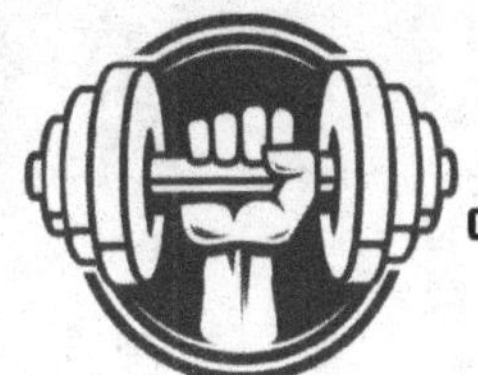

NAME:

GOALS:

DATE:

STATS:

WEIGHT:

EXERCISE:	SETS	REPS	WEIGHT	REST	SETS	REPS	WEIGHT	REST	SETS	REPS	WEIGHT	REST	SETS	REPS	WEIGHT	REST

CARDIO:	TIME	DIST.	INT.	PACE	TIME	DIST.	INT.	PACE	TIME	DIST.	INT.	PACE	TIME	DIST.	INT.	PACE

WORKOUT LOG

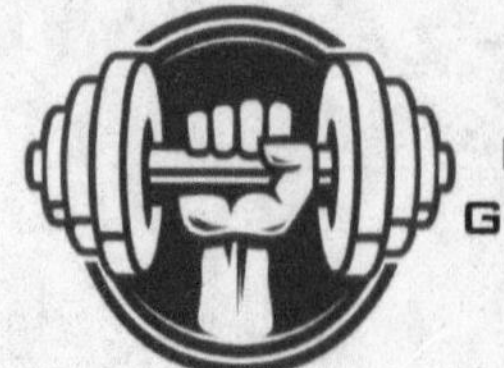

NAME:

GOALS:

DATE:

STATS:

WEIGHT:

EXERCISE:	SETS	REPS	WEIGHT	REST	SETS	REPS	WEIGHT	REST	SETS	REPS	WEIGHT	REST	SETS	REPS	WEIGHT	REST

CARDIO:	TIME	DIST.	INT.	PACE	TIME	DIST.	INT.	PACE	TIME	DIST.	INT.	PACE	TIME	DIST.	INT.	PACE

WORKOUT LOG

NAME:
GOALS:
DATE:
STATS:
WEIGHT:

EXERCISE:	SETS	REPS	WEIGHT	REST	SETS	REPS	WEIGHT	REST	SETS	REPS	WEIGHT	REST	SETS	REPS	WEIGHT	REST

CARDIO:	TIME	DIST.	INT.	PACE	TIME	DIST.	INT.	PACE	TIME	DIST.	INT.	PACE	TIME	DIST.	INT.	PACE

WORKOUT LOG

NAME:

GOALS:

DATE:

STATS:

WEIGHT:

EXERCISE:	SETS	REPS	WEIGHT	REST	SETS	REPS	WEIGHT	REST	SETS	REPS	WEIGHT	REST	SETS	REPS	WEIGHT	REST

CARDIO:	TIME	DIST.	INT.	PACE	TIME	DIST.	INT.	PACE	TIME	DIST.	INT.	PACE	TIME	DIST.	INT.	PACE

WORKOUT LOG

NAME:
GOALS:
DATE:
STATS:
WEIGHT:

EXERCISE:	SETS	REPS	WEIGHT	REST	SETS	REPS	WEIGHT	REST	SETS	REPS	WEIGHT	REST	SETS	REPS	WEIGHT	REST

CARDIO:	TIME	DIST.	INT.	PACE	TIME	DIST.	INT.	PACE	TIME	DIST.	INT.	PACE	TIME	DIST.	INT.	PACE

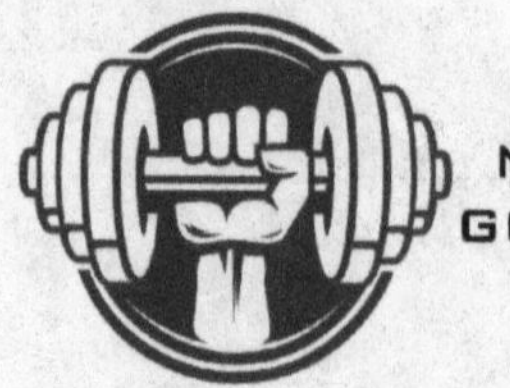

WORKOUT LOG

NAME:

GOALS:

DATE:

STATS:

WEIGHT:

EXERCISE:	SETS	REPS	WEIGHT	REST	SETS	REPS	WEIGHT	REST	SETS	REPS	WEIGHT	REST	SETS	REPS	WEIGHT	REST

CARDIO:	TIME	DIST.	INT.	PACE	TIME	DIST.	INT.	PACE	TIME	DIST.	INT.	PACE	TIME	DIST.	INT.	PACE

WORKOUT LOG

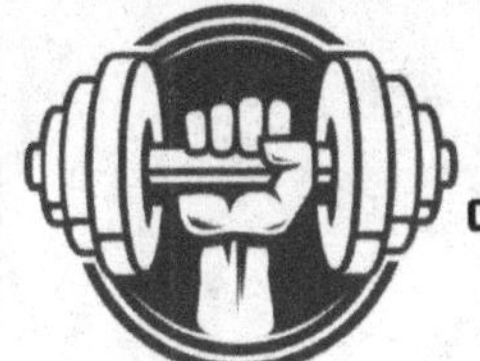

NAME:

GOALS:

DATE:

STATS:

WEIGHT:

EXERCISE:	SETS	REPS	WEIGHT	REST	SETS	REPS	WEIGHT	REST	SETS	REPS	WEIGHT	REST	SETS	REPS	WEIGHT	REST

CARDIO:	TIME	DIST.	INT.	PACE	TIME	DIST.	INT.	PACE	TIME	DIST.	INT.	PACE	TIME	DIST.	INT.	PACE

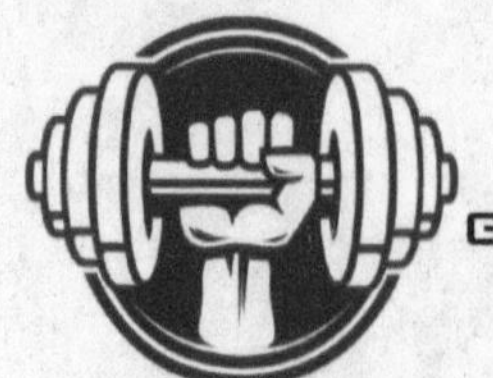

WORKOUT LOG

NAME:
GOALS:
DATE:
STATS:
WEIGHT:

EXERCISE:	SETS	REPS	WEIGHT	REST	SETS	REPS	WEIGHT	REST	SETS	REPS	WEIGHT	REST	SETS	REPS	WEIGHT	REST

CARDIO:	TIME	DIST.	INT.	PACE	TIME	DIST.	INT.	PACE	TIME	DIST.	INT.	PACE	TIME	DIST.	INT.	PACE

WORKOUT LOG

NAME:

GOALS:

DATE:

STATS:

WEIGHT:

EXERCISE:	SETS	REPS	WEIGHT	REST	SETS	REPS	WEIGHT	REST	SETS	REPS	WEIGHT	REST	SETS	REPS	WEIGHT	REST

CARDIO:	TIME	DIST.	INT.	PACE	TIME	DIST.	INT.	PACE	TIME	DIST.	INT.	PACE	TIME	DIST.	INT.	PACE

WORKOUT LOG

NAME:

GOALS:

DATE:

STATS:

WEIGHT:

EXERCISE:	SETS	REPS	WEIGHT	REST	SETS	REPS	WEIGHT	REST	SETS	REPS	WEIGHT	REST	SETS	REPS	WEIGHT	REST

CARDIO:	TIME	DIST.	INT.	PACE	TIME	DIST.	INT.	PACE	TIME	DIST.	INT.	PACE	TIME	DIST.	INT.	PACE

WORKOUT LOG

NAME:

GOALS:

DATE:

STATS:

WEIGHT:

EXERCISE:	SETS	REPS	WEIGHT	REST	SETS	REPS	WEIGHT	REST	SETS	REPS	WEIGHT	REST	SETS	REPS	WEIGHT	REST

CARDIO:	TIME	DIST.	INT.	PACE	TIME	DIST.	INT.	PACE	TIME	DIST.	INT.	PACE	TIME	DIST.	INT.	PACE

WORKOUT LOG

NAME:

GOALS:

DATE:

STATS:

WEIGHT:

EXERCISE:	SETS	REPS	WEIGHT	REST	SETS	REPS	WEIGHT	REST	SETS	REPS	WEIGHT	REST	SETS	REPS	WEIGHT	REST

CARDIO:	TIME	DIST.	INT.	PACE	TIME	DIST.	INT.	PACE	TIME	DIST.	INT.	PACE	TIME	DIST.	INT.	PACE

WORKOUT LOG

NAME:

GOALS:

DATE:

STATS:

WEIGHT:

EXERCISE:	SETS	REPS	WEIGHT	REST	SETS	REPS	WEIGHT	REST	SETS	REPS	WEIGHT	REST	SETS	REPS	WEIGHT	REST

CARDIO:	TIME	DIST.	INT.	PACE	TIME	DIST.	INT.	PACE	TIME	DIST.	INT.	PACE	TIME	DIST.	INT.	PACE

WORKOUT LOG

NAME:

GOALS:

DATE:

STATS:

WEIGHT:

EXERCISE:	SETS	REPS	WEIGHT	REST	SETS	REPS	WEIGHT	REST	SETS	REPS	WEIGHT	REST	SETS	REPS	WEIGHT	REST

CARDIO:	TIME	DIST.	INT.	PACE	TIME	DIST.	INT.	PACE	TIME	DIST.	INT.	PACE	TIME	DIST.	INT.	PACE

WORKOUT LOG

NAME:

GOALS:

DATE:

STATS:

WEIGHT:

EXERCISE:	SETS	REPS	WEIGHT	REST	SETS	REPS	WEIGHT	REST	SETS	REPS	WEIGHT	REST	SETS	REPS	WEIGHT	REST

CARDIO:	TIME	DIST.	INT.	PACE	TIME	DIST.	INT.	PACE	TIME	DIST.	INT.	PACE	TIME	DIST.	INT.	PACE

WORKOUT LOG

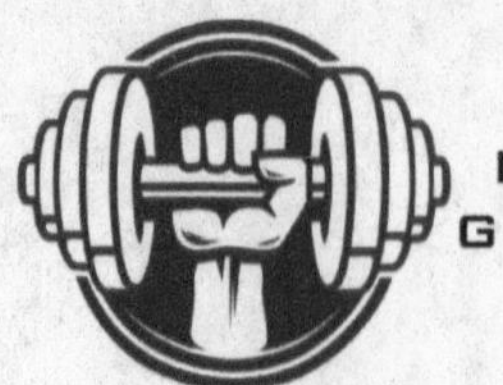

NAME:

GOALS:

DATE:

STATS:

WEIGHT:

EXERCISE:	SETS	REPS	WEIGHT	REST	SETS	REPS	WEIGHT	REST	SETS	REPS	WEIGHT	REST	SETS	REPS	WEIGHT	REST

CARDIO:	TIME	DIST.	INT.	PACE	TIME	DIST.	INT.	PACE	TIME	DIST.	INT.	PACE	TIME	DIST.	INT.	PACE

WORKOUT LOG

NAME:

GOALS:

DATE:

STATS:

WEIGHT:

EXERCISE:	SETS	REPS	WEIGHT	REST	SETS	REPS	WEIGHT	REST	SETS	REPS	WEIGHT	REST	SETS	REPS	WEIGHT	REST

CARDIO:	TIME	DIST.	INT.	PACE	TIME	DIST.	INT.	PACE	TIME	DIST.	INT.	PACE	TIME	DIST.	INT.	PACE

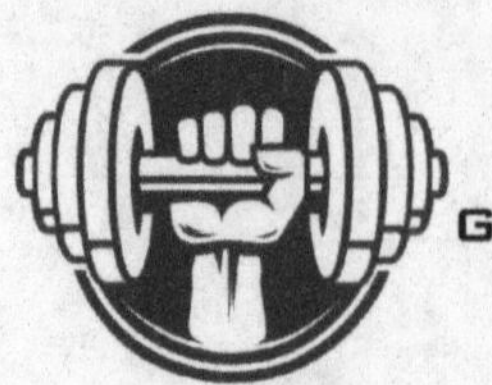

WORKOUT LOG

NAME:

GOALS:

DATE:

STATS:

WEIGHT:

EXERCISE:	SETS	REPS	WEIGHT	REST	SETS	REPS	WEIGHT	REST	SETS	REPS	WEIGHT	REST	SETS	REPS	WEIGHT	REST

CARDIO:	TIME	DIST.	INT.	PACE	TIME	DIST.	INT.	PACE	TIME	DIST.	INT.	PACE	TIME	DIST.	INT.	PACE

WORKOUT LOG

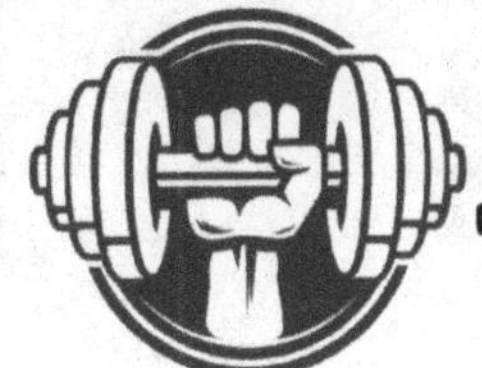

NAME:

GOALS:

DATE:

STATS:

WEIGHT:

EXERCISE:	SETS	REPS	WEIGHT	REST	SETS	REPS	WEIGHT	REST	SETS	REPS	WEIGHT	REST	SETS	REPS	WEIGHT	REST

CARDIO:	TIME	DIST.	INT.	PACE	TIME	DIST.	INT.	PACE	TIME	DIST.	INT.	PACE	TIME	DIST.	INT.	PACE

WORKOUT LOG

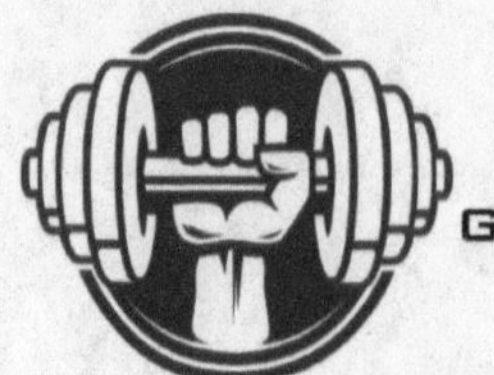

NAME:

GOALS:

DATE:

STATS:

WEIGHT:

EXERCISE:	SETS	REPS	WEIGHT	REST	SETS	REPS	WEIGHT	REST	SETS	REPS	WEIGHT	REST	SETS	REPS	WEIGHT	REST

CARDIO:	TIME	DIST.	INT.	PACE	TIME	DIST.	INT.	PACE	TIME	DIST.	INT.	PACE	TIME	DIST.	INT.	PACE

WORKOUT LOG

NAME: _______________________________

GOALS: _______________________________

DATE: _______________________________

STATS: _______________________________

WEIGHT: _______________________________

EXERCISE:	SETS	REPS	WEIGHT	REST	SETS	REPS	WEIGHT	REST	SETS	REPS	WEIGHT	REST	SETS	REPS	WEIGHT	REST

CARDIO:	TIME	DIST.	INT.	PACE	TIME	DIST.	INT.	PACE	TIME	DIST.	INT.	PACE	TIME	DIST.	INT.	PACE

WORKOUT LOG

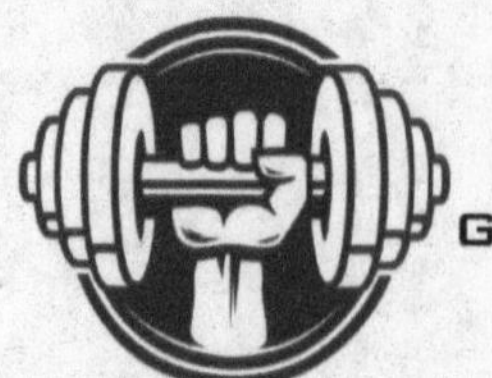

NAME:

GOALS:

DATE:

STATS:

WEIGHT:

EXERCISE:	SETS	REPS	WEIGHT	REST	SETS	REPS	WEIGHT	REST	SETS	REPS	WEIGHT	REST	SETS	REPS	WEIGHT	REST

CARDIO:	TIME	DIST.	INT.	PACE	TIME	DIST.	INT.	PACE	TIME	DIST.	INT.	PACE	TIME	DIST.	INT.	PACE

WORKOUT LOG

NAME:
GOALS:
DATE:
STATS:
WEIGHT:

EXERCISE:	SETS	REPS	WEIGHT	REST	SETS	REPS	WEIGHT	REST	SETS	REPS	WEIGHT	REST	SETS	REPS	WEIGHT	REST

CARDIO:	TIME	DIST.	INT.	PACE	TIME	DIST.	INT.	PACE	TIME	DIST.	INT.	PACE	TIME	DIST.	INT.	PACE

WORKOUT LOG

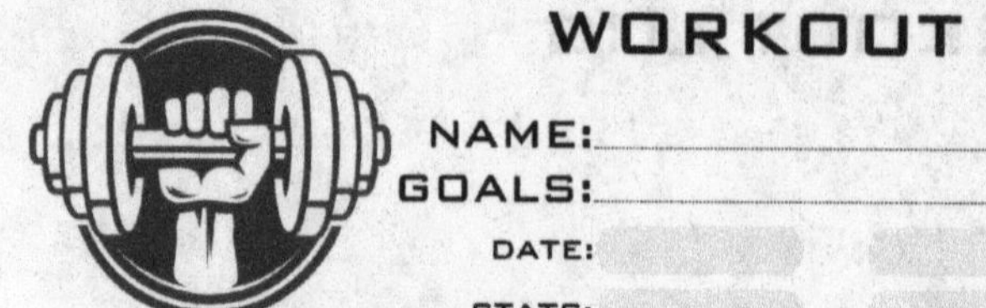

NAME:

GOALS:

DATE:

STATS:

WEIGHT:

EXERCISE:	SETS	REPS	WEIGHT	REST	SETS	REPS	WEIGHT	REST	SETS	REPS	WEIGHT	REST	SETS	REPS	WEIGHT	REST

CARDIO:	TIME	DIST.	INT.	PACE	TIME	DIST.	INT.	PACE	TIME	DIST.	INT.	PACE	TIME	DIST.	INT.	PACE

WORKOUT LOG

NAME:
GOALS:
DATE:
STATS:
WEIGHT:

EXERCISE:	SETS	REPS	WEIGHT	REST	SETS	REPS	WEIGHT	REST	SETS	REPS	WEIGHT	REST	SETS	REPS	WEIGHT	REST

CARDIO:	TIME	DIST.	INT.	PACE	TIME	DIST.	INT.	PACE	TIME	DIST.	INT.	PACE	TIME	DIST.	INT.	PACE

WORKOUT LOG

NAME:

GOALS:

DATE:

STATS:

WEIGHT:

EXERCISE:	SETS	REPS	WEIGHT	REST	SETS	REPS	WEIGHT	REST	SETS	REPS	WEIGHT	REST	SETS	REPS	WEIGHT	REST

CARDIO:	TIME	DIST.	INT.	PACE	TIME	DIST.	INT.	PACE	TIME	DIST.	INT.	PACE	TIME	DIST.	INT.	PACE

WORKOUT LOG

NAME:

GOALS:

DATE:

STATS:

WEIGHT:

EXERCISE:	SETS	REPS	WEIGHT	REST	SETS	REPS	WEIGHT	REST	SETS	REPS	WEIGHT	REST	SETS	REPS	WEIGHT	REST

CARDIO:	TIME	DIST.	INT.	PACE	TIME	DIST.	INT.	PACE	TIME	DIST.	INT.	PACE	TIME	DIST.	INT.	PACE

WORKOUT LOG

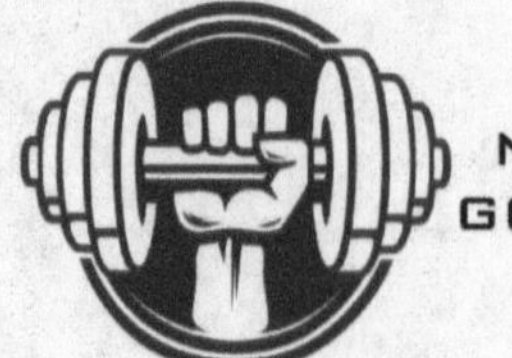

NAME:

GOALS:

DATE:

STATS:

WEIGHT:

EXERCISE:	SETS	REPS	WEIGHT	REST	SETS	REPS	WEIGHT	REST	SETS	REPS	WEIGHT	REST	SETS	REPS	WEIGHT	REST

CARDIO:	TIME	DIST.	INT.	PACE	TIME	DIST.	INT.	PACE	TIME	DIST.	INT.	PACE	TIME	DIST.	INT.	PACE

WORKOUT LOG

NAME:

GOALS:

DATE:

STATS:

WEIGHT:

EXERCISE:	SETS	REPS	WEIGHT	REST	SETS	REPS	WEIGHT	REST	SETS	REPS	WEIGHT	REST	SETS	REPS	WEIGHT	REST

CARDIO:	TIME	DIST.	INT.	PACE	TIME	DIST.	INT.	PACE	TIME	DIST.	INT.	PACE	TIME	DIST.	INT.	PACE

WORKOUT LOG

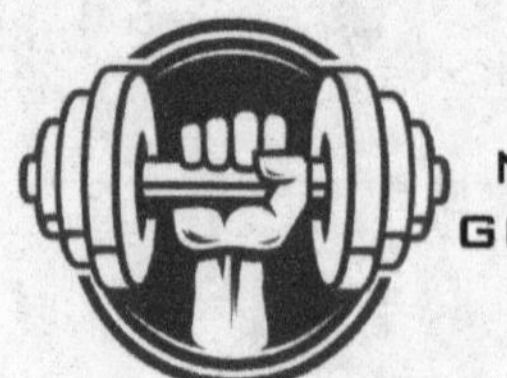

NAME:

GOALS:

DATE:

STATS:

WEIGHT:

EXERCISE:	SETS	REPS	WEIGHT	REST	SETS	REPS	WEIGHT	REST	SETS	REPS	WEIGHT	REST	SETS	REPS	WEIGHT	REST

CARDIO:	TIME	DIST.	INT.	PACE	TIME	DIST.	INT.	PACE	TIME	DIST.	INT.	PACE	TIME	DIST.	INT.	PACE

WORKOUT LOG

NAME: _______________________________

GOALS: _______________________________

DATE:

STATS:

WEIGHT:

EXERCISE:	SETS	REPS	WEIGHT	REST	SETS	REPS	WEIGHT	REST	SETS	REPS	WEIGHT	REST	SETS	REPS	WEIGHT	REST

CARDIO:	TIME	DIST.	INT.	PACE	TIME	DIST.	INT.	PACE	TIME	DIST.	INT.	PACE	TIME	DIST.	INT.	PACE

WORKOUT LOG

NAME:
GOALS:
DATE:
STATS:
WEIGHT:

EXERCISE:	SETS	REPS	WEIGHT	REST	SETS	REPS	WEIGHT	REST	SETS	REPS	WEIGHT	REST	SETS	REPS	WEIGHT	REST

CARDIO:	TIME	DIST.	INT.	PACE	TIME	DIST.	INT.	PACE	TIME	DIST.	INT.	PACE	TIME	DIST.	INT.	PACE

WORKOUT LOG

NAME:
GOALS:
DATE:
STATS:
WEIGHT:

EXERCISE:	SETS	REPS	WEIGHT	REST	SETS	REPS	WEIGHT	REST	SETS	REPS	WEIGHT	REST	SETS	REPS	WEIGHT	REST

CARDIO:	TIME	DIST.	INT.	PACE	TIME	DIST.	INT.	PACE	TIME	DIST.	INT.	PACE	TIME	DIST.	INT.	PACE

WORKOUT LOG

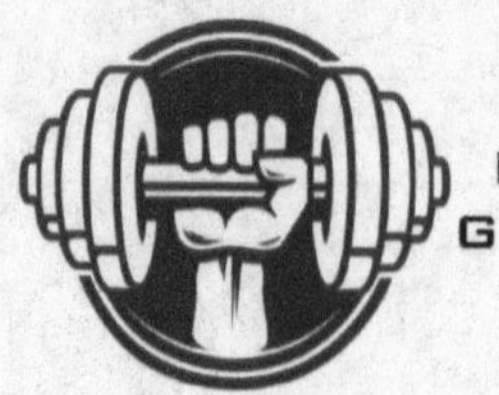

NAME:

GOALS:

DATE:

STATS:

WEIGHT:

EXERCISE:	SETS	REPS	WEIGHT	REST	SETS	REPS	WEIGHT	REST	SETS	REPS	WEIGHT	REST	SETS	REPS	WEIGHT	REST

CARDIO:	TIME	DIST.	INT.	PACE	TIME	DIST.	INT.	PACE	TIME	DIST.	INT.	PACE	TIME	DIST.	INT.	PACE

WORKOUT LOG

NAME:

GOALS:

DATE:

STATS:

WEIGHT:

EXERCISE:	SETS	REPS	WEIGHT	REST	SETS	REPS	WEIGHT	REST	SETS	REPS	WEIGHT	REST	SETS	REPS	WEIGHT	REST

CARDIO:	TIME	DIST.	INT.	PACE	TIME	DIST.	INT.	PACE	TIME	DIST.	INT.	PACE	TIME	DIST.	INT.	PACE

WORKOUT LOG

NAME:

GOALS:

DATE:

STATS:

WEIGHT:

EXERCISE:	SETS	REPS	WEIGHT	REST	SETS	REPS	WEIGHT	REST	SETS	REPS	WEIGHT	REST	SETS	REPS	WEIGHT	REST

CARDIO:	TIME	DIST.	INT.	PACE	TIME	DIST.	INT.	PACE	TIME	DIST.	INT.	PACE	TIME	DIST.	INT.	PACE

WORKOUT LOG

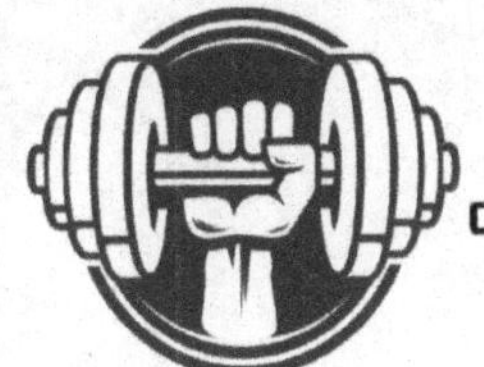

NAME:

GOALS:

DATE:

STATS:

WEIGHT:

EXERCISE:	SETS	REPS	WEIGHT	REST	SETS	REPS	WEIGHT	REST	SETS	REPS	WEIGHT	REST	SETS	REPS	WEIGHT	REST

CARDIO:	TIME	DIST.	INT.	PACE	TIME	DIST.	INT.	PACE	TIME	DIST.	INT.	PACE	TIME	DIST.	INT.	PACE

WORKOUT LOG

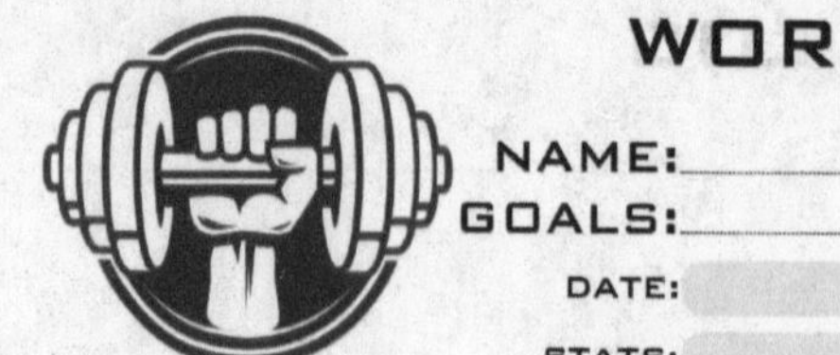

NAME:

GOALS:

DATE:

STATS:

WEIGHT:

EXERCISE:	SETS	REPS	WEIGHT	REST	SETS	REPS	WEIGHT	REST	SETS	REPS	WEIGHT	REST	SETS	REPS	WEIGHT	REST

CARDIO:	TIME	DIST.	INT.	PACE	TIME	DIST.	INT.	PACE	TIME	DIST.	INT.	PACE	TIME	DIST.	INT.	PACE

WORKOUT LOG

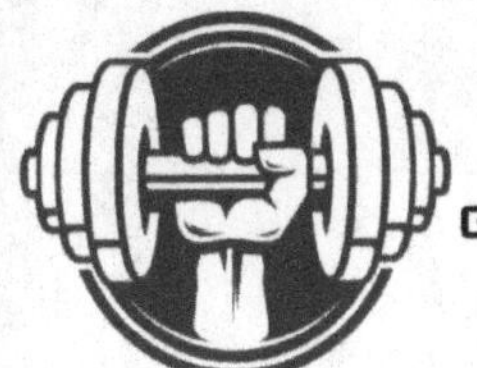

NAME:

GOALS:

DATE:

STATS:

WEIGHT:

EXERCISE:	SETS	REPS	WEIGHT	REST	SETS	REPS	WEIGHT	REST	SETS	REPS	WEIGHT	REST	SETS	REPS	WEIGHT	REST

CARDIO:	TIME	DIST.	INT.	PACE	TIME	DIST.	INT.	PACE	TIME	DIST.	INT.	PACE	TIME	DIST.	INT.	PACE

WORKOUT LOG

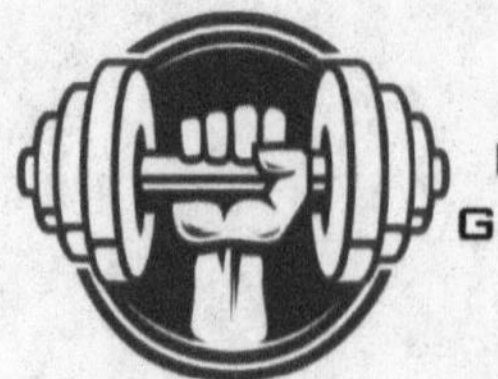

NAME:

GOALS:

DATE:

STATS:

WEIGHT:

EXERCISE:

Exercise	SETS	REPS	WEIGHT	REST	SETS	REPS	WEIGHT	REST	SETS	REPS	WEIGHT	REST	SETS	REPS	WEIGHT	REST

CARDIO:

Cardio	TIME	DIST.	INT.	PACE	TIME	DIST.	INT.	PACE	TIME	DIST.	INT.	PACE	TIME	DIST.	INT.	PACE

WORKOUT LOG

NAME:

GOALS:

DATE:

STATS:

WEIGHT:

EXERCISE:	SETS	REPS	WEIGHT	REST	SETS	REPS	WEIGHT	REST	SETS	REPS	WEIGHT	REST	SETS	REPS	WEIGHT	REST

CARDIO:	TIME	DIST.	INT.	PACE	TIME	DIST.	INT.	PACE	TIME	DIST.	INT.	PACE	TIME	DIST.	INT.	PACE

WORKOUT LOG

NAME:

GOALS:

DATE:

STATS:

WEIGHT:

EXERCISE:	SETS	REPS	WEIGHT	REST	SETS	REPS	WEIGHT	REST	SETS	REPS	WEIGHT	REST	SETS	REPS	WEIGHT	REST

CARDIO:	TIME	DIST.	INT.	PACE	TIME	DIST.	INT.	PACE	TIME	DIST.	INT.	PACE	TIME	DIST.	INT.	PACE

WORKOUT LOG

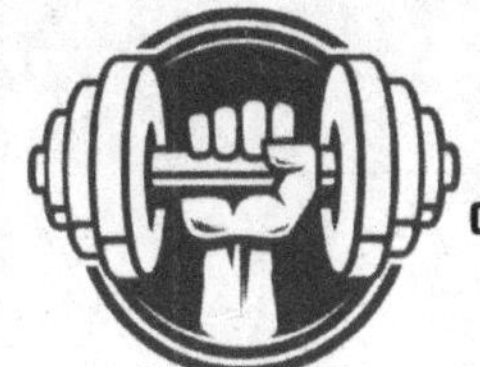

NAME:

GOALS:

DATE:

STATS:

WEIGHT:

EXERCISE:	SETS	REPS	WEIGHT	REST	SETS	REPS	WEIGHT	REST	SETS	REPS	WEIGHT	REST	SETS	REPS	WEIGHT	REST

CARDIO:	TIME	DIST.	INT.	PACE	TIME	DIST.	INT.	PACE	TIME	DIST.	INT.	PACE	TIME	DIST.	INT.	PACE

WORKOUT LOG

NAME:

GOALS:

DATE:

STATS:

WEIGHT:

EXERCISE:	SETS	REPS	WEIGHT	REST	SETS	REPS	WEIGHT	REST	SETS	REPS	WEIGHT	REST	SETS	REPS	WEIGHT	REST

CARDIO:	TIME	DIST.	INT.	PACE	TIME	DIST.	INT.	PACE	TIME	DIST.	INT.	PACE	TIME	DIST.	INT.	PACE

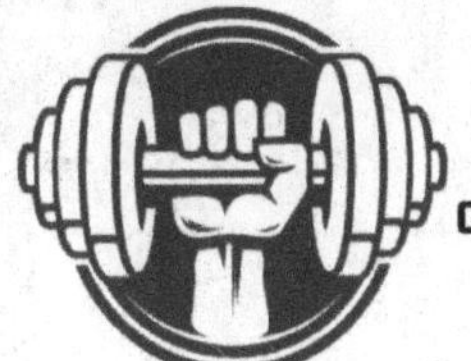

WORKOUT LOG

NAME:

GOALS:

DATE:

STATS:

WEIGHT:

EXERCISE:	SETS	REPS	WEIGHT	REST	SETS	REPS	WEIGHT	REST	SETS	REPS	WEIGHT	REST	SETS	REPS	WEIGHT	REST

CARDIO:	TIME	DIST.	INT.	PACE	TIME	DIST.	INT.	PACE	TIME	DIST.	INT.	PACE	TIME	DIST.	INT.	PACE

WORKOUT LOG

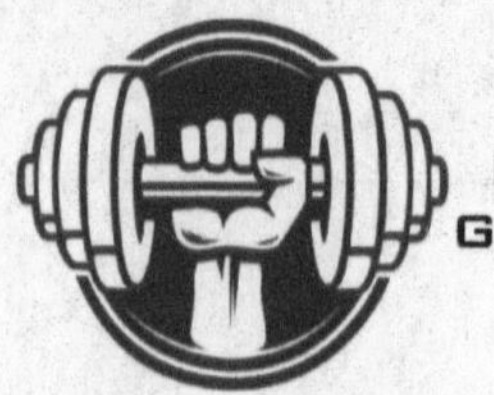

NAME:

GOALS:

DATE:

STATS:

WEIGHT:

EXERCISE:	SETS	REPS	WEIGHT	REST	SETS	REPS	WEIGHT	REST	SETS	REPS	WEIGHT	REST	SETS	REPS	WEIGHT	REST

CARDIO:	TIME	DIST.	INT.	PACE	TIME	DIST.	INT.	PACE	TIME	DIST.	INT.	PACE	TIME	DIST.	INT.	PACE

WORKOUT LOG

NAME:
GOALS:
DATE:
STATS:
WEIGHT:

EXERCISE:	SETS	REPS	WEIGHT	REST	SETS	REPS	WEIGHT	REST	SETS	REPS	WEIGHT	REST	SETS	REPS	WEIGHT	REST

CARDIO:	TIME	DIST.	INT.	PACE	TIME	DIST.	INT.	PACE	TIME	DIST.	INT.	PACE	TIME	DIST.	INT.	PACE

WORKOUT LOG

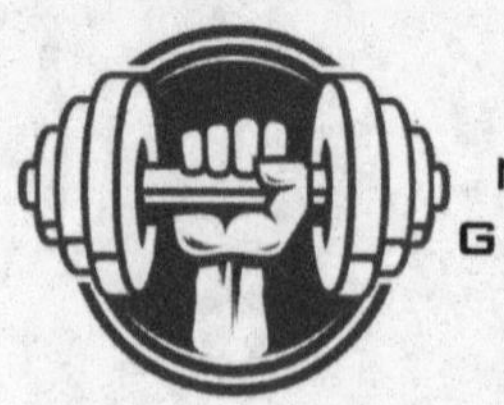

NAME:

GOALS:

DATE:

STATS:

WEIGHT:

EXERCISE:	SETS	REPS	WEIGHT	REST	SETS	REPS	WEIGHT	REST	SETS	REPS	WEIGHT	REST	SETS	REPS	WEIGHT	REST

CARDIO:	TIME	DIST.	INT.	PACE	TIME	DIST.	INT.	PACE	TIME	DIST.	INT.	PACE	TIME	DIST.	INT.	PACE

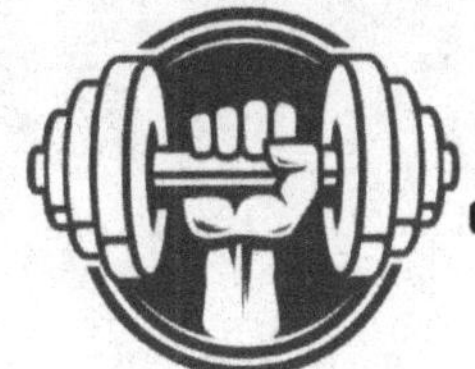

WORKOUT LOG

NAME:
GOALS:
DATE:
STATS:
WEIGHT:

EXERCISE:	SETS	REPS	WEIGHT	REST	SETS	REPS	WEIGHT	REST	SETS	REPS	WEIGHT	REST	SETS	REPS	WEIGHT	REST

CARDIO:	TIME	DIST.	INT.	PACE	TIME	DIST.	INT.	PACE	TIME	DIST.	INT.	PACE	TIME	DIST.	INT.	PACE

WORKOUT LOG

NAME:

GOALS:

DATE:

STATS:

WEIGHT:

EXERCISE:	SETS	REPS	WEIGHT	REST	SETS	REPS	WEIGHT	REST	SETS	REPS	WEIGHT	REST	SETS	REPS	WEIGHT	REST

CARDIO:	TIME	DIST.	INT.	PACE	TIME	DIST.	INT.	PACE	TIME	DIST.	INT.	PACE	TIME	DIST.	INT.	PACE

WORKOUT LOG

NAME:

GOALS:

DATE:

STATS:

WEIGHT:

EXERCISE:	SETS	REPS	WEIGHT	REST	SETS	REPS	WEIGHT	REST	SETS	REPS	WEIGHT	REST	SETS	REPS	WEIGHT	REST

CARDIO:	TIME	DIST.	INT.	PACE	TIME	DIST.	INT.	PACE	TIME	DIST.	INT.	PACE	TIME	DIST.	INT.	PACE

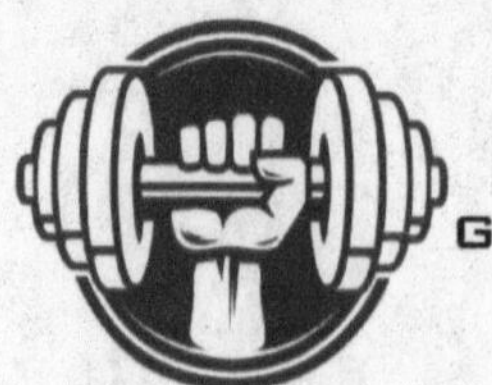

WORKOUT LOG

NAME:
GOALS:
DATE:
STATS:
WEIGHT:

EXERCISE:	SETS	REPS	WEIGHT	REST	SETS	REPS	WEIGHT	REST	SETS	REPS	WEIGHT	REST	SETS	REPS	WEIGHT	REST

CARDIO:	TIME	DIST.	INT.	PACE	TIME	DIST.	INT.	PACE	TIME	DIST.	INT.	PACE	TIME	DIST.	INT.	PACE

WORKOUT LOG

NAME:

GOALS:

DATE:

STATS:

WEIGHT:

EXERCISE:	SETS	REPS	WEIGHT	REST	SETS	REPS	WEIGHT	REST	SETS	REPS	WEIGHT	REST	SETS	REPS	WEIGHT	REST

CARDIO:	TIME	DIST.	INT.	PACE	TIME	DIST.	INT.	PACE	TIME	DIST.	INT.	PACE	TIME	DIST.	INT.	PACE

WORKOUT LOG

NAME:

GOALS:

DATE:

STATS:

WEIGHT:

EXERCISE:	SETS	REPS	WEIGHT	REST	SETS	REPS	WEIGHT	REST	SETS	REPS	WEIGHT	REST	SETS	REPS	WEIGHT	REST

CARDIO:	TIME	DIST.	INT.	PACE	TIME	DIST.	INT.	PACE	TIME	DIST.	INT.	PACE	TIME	DIST.	INT.	PACE

WORKOUT LOG

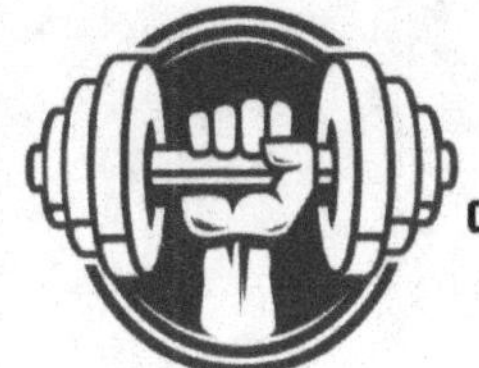

NAME:

GOALS:

DATE:

STATS:

WEIGHT:

EXERCISE:	SETS	REPS	WEIGHT	REST	SETS	REPS	WEIGHT	REST	SETS	REPS	WEIGHT	REST	SETS	REPS	WEIGHT	REST

CARDIO:	TIME	DIST.	INT.	PACE	TIME	DIST.	INT.	PACE	TIME	DIST.	INT.	PACE	TIME	DIST.	INT.	PACE

WORKOUT LOG

NAME:

GOALS:

DATE:

STATS:

WEIGHT:

EXERCISE:	SETS	REPS	WEIGHT	REST	SETS	REPS	WEIGHT	REST	SETS	REPS	WEIGHT	REST	SETS	REPS	WEIGHT	REST

CARDIO:	TIME	DIST.	INT.	PACE	TIME	DIST.	INT.	PACE	TIME	DIST.	INT.	PACE	TIME	DIST.	INT.	PACE

WORKOUT LOG

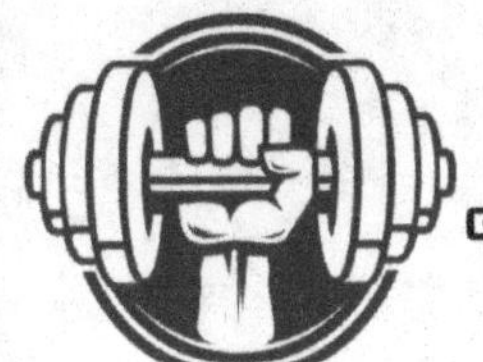

NAME:

GOALS:

DATE:

STATS:

WEIGHT:

EXERCISE:	SETS	REPS	WEIGHT	REST	SETS	REPS	WEIGHT	REST	SETS	REPS	WEIGHT	REST	SETS	REPS	WEIGHT	REST

CARDIO:	TIME	DIST.	INT.	PACE	TIME	DIST.	INT.	PACE	TIME	DIST.	INT.	PACE	TIME	DIST.	INT.	PACE

WORKOUT LOG

NAME:

GOALS:

DATE:

STATS:

WEIGHT:

EXERCISE:	SETS	REPS	WEIGHT	REST	SETS	REPS	WEIGHT	REST	SETS	REPS	WEIGHT	REST	SETS	REPS	WEIGHT	REST

CARDIO:	TIME	DIST.	INT.	PACE	TIME	DIST.	INT.	PACE	TIME	DIST.	INT.	PACE	TIME	DIST.	INT.	PACE

WORKOUT LOG

NAME:

GOALS:

DATE:

STATS:

WEIGHT:

EXERCISE:	SETS	REPS	WEIGHT	REST	SETS	REPS	WEIGHT	REST	SETS	REPS	WEIGHT	REST	SETS	REPS	WEIGHT	REST

CARDIO:	TIME	DIST.	INT.	PACE	TIME	DIST.	INT.	PACE	TIME	DIST.	INT.	PACE	TIME	DIST.	INT.	PACE

WORKOUT LOG

NAME:

GOALS:

DATE:

STATS:

WEIGHT:

EXERCISE:	SETS	REPS	WEIGHT	REST	SETS	REPS	WEIGHT	REST	SETS	REPS	WEIGHT	REST	SETS	REPS	WEIGHT	REST

CARDIO:	TIME	DIST.	INT.	PACE	TIME	DIST.	INT.	PACE	TIME	DIST.	INT.	PACE	TIME	DIST.	INT.	PACE

WORKOUT LOG

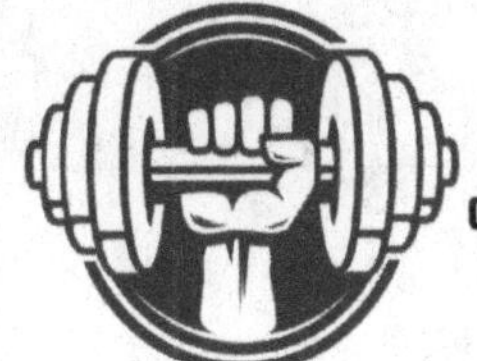

NAME:

GOALS:

DATE:

STATS:

WEIGHT:

EXERCISE:	SETS	REPS	WEIGHT	REST	SETS	REPS	WEIGHT	REST	SETS	REPS	WEIGHT	REST	SETS	REPS	WEIGHT	REST

CARDIO:	TIME	DIST.	INT.	PACE	TIME	DIST.	INT.	PACE	TIME	DIST.	INT.	PACE	TIME	DIST.	INT.	PACE

WORKOUT LOG

NAME: _______________________________

GOALS: _______________________________

DATE:

STATS:

WEIGHT:

EXERCISE:	SETS	REPS	WEIGHT	REST	SETS	REPS	WEIGHT	REST	SETS	REPS	WEIGHT	REST	SETS	REPS	WEIGHT	REST

CARDIO:	TIME	DIST.	INT.	PACE	TIME	DIST.	INT.	PACE	TIME	DIST.	INT.	PACE	TIME	DIST.	INT.	PACE

WORKOUT LOG

NAME:
GOALS:
DATE:
STATS:
WEIGHT:

EXERCISE:	SETS	REPS	WEIGHT	REST	SETS	REPS	WEIGHT	REST	SETS	REPS	WEIGHT	REST	SETS	REPS	WEIGHT	REST

CARDIO:	TIME	DIST.	INT.	PACE	TIME	DIST.	INT.	PACE	TIME	DIST.	INT.	PACE	TIME	DIST.	INT.	PACE

WORKOUT LOG

NAME:
GOALS:
DATE:
STATS:
WEIGHT:

EXERCISE:	SETS	REPS	WEIGHT	REST	SETS	REPS	WEIGHT	REST	SETS	REPS	WEIGHT	REST	SETS	REPS	WEIGHT	REST

CARDIO:	TIME	DIST.	INT.	PACE	TIME	DIST.	INT.	PACE	TIME	DIST.	INT.	PACE	TIME	DIST.	INT.	PACE

WORKOUT LOG

NAME: ____

GOALS: ____

DATE:

STATS:

WEIGHT:

EXERCISE:	SETS	REPS	WEIGHT	REST	SETS	REPS	WEIGHT	REST	SETS	REPS	WEIGHT	REST	SETS	REPS	WEIGHT	REST

CARDIO:	TIME	DIST.	INT.	PACE	TIME	DIST.	INT.	PACE	TIME	DIST.	INT.	PACE	TIME	DIST.	INT.	PACE

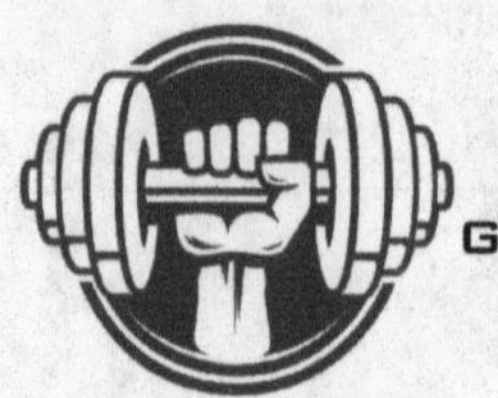

WORKOUT LOG

NAME:

GOALS:

DATE:

STATS:

WEIGHT:

EXERCISE:	SETS	REPS	WEIGHT	REST	SETS	REPS	WEIGHT	REST	SETS	REPS	WEIGHT	REST	SETS	REPS	WEIGHT	REST

CARDIO:	TIME	DIST.	INT.	PACE	TIME	DIST.	INT.	PACE	TIME	DIST.	INT.	PACE	TIME	DIST.	INT.	PACE

WORKOUT LOG

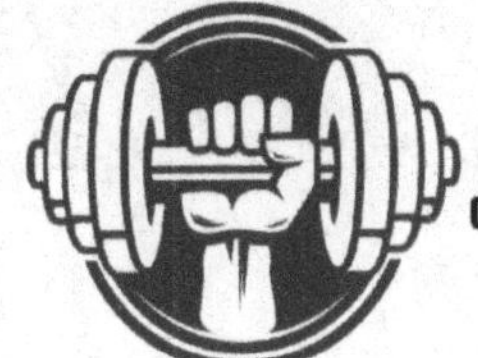

NAME:

GOALS:

DATE:

STATS:

WEIGHT:

EXERCISE:	SETS	REPS	WEIGHT	REST	SETS	REPS	WEIGHT	REST	SETS	REPS	WEIGHT	REST	SETS	REPS	WEIGHT	REST

CARDIO:	TIME	DIST.	INT.	PACE	TIME	DIST.	INT.	PACE	TIME	DIST.	INT.	PACE	TIME	DIST.	INT.	PACE

WORKOUT LOG

NAME:

GOALS:

DATE:

STATS:

WEIGHT:

EXERCISE:	SETS	REPS	WEIGHT	REST	SETS	REPS	WEIGHT	REST	SETS	REPS	WEIGHT	REST	SETS	REPS	WEIGHT	REST

CARDIO:	TIME	DIST.	INT.	PACE	TIME	DIST.	INT.	PACE	TIME	DIST.	INT.	PACE	TIME	DIST.	INT.	PACE

WORKOUT LOG

NAME: ___________________________
GOALS: ___________________________
DATE: ___________
STATS: ___________
WEIGHT: ___________

EXERCISE:	SETS	REPS	WEIGHT	REST	SETS	REPS	WEIGHT	REST	SETS	REPS	WEIGHT	REST	SETS	REPS	WEIGHT	REST

CARDIO:	TIME	DIST.	INT.	PACE	TIME	DIST.	INT.	PACE	TIME	DIST.	INT.	PACE	TIME	DIST.	INT.	PACE

WORKOUT LOG

NAME:

GOALS:

DATE:

STATS:

WEIGHT:

EXERCISE:	SETS	REPS	WEIGHT	REST	SETS	REPS	WEIGHT	REST	SETS	REPS	WEIGHT	REST	SETS	REPS	WEIGHT	REST

CARDIO:	TIME	DIST.	INT.	PACE	TIME	DIST.	INT.	PACE	TIME	DIST.	INT.	PACE	TIME	DIST.	INT.	PACE

WORKOUT LOG

NAME:

GOALS:

DATE:

STATS:

WEIGHT:

EXERCISE:	SETS	REPS	WEIGHT	REST	SETS	REPS	WEIGHT	REST	SETS	REPS	WEIGHT	REST	SETS	REPS	WEIGHT	REST

CARDIO:	TIME	DIST.	INT.	PACE	TIME	DIST.	INT.	PACE	TIME	DIST.	INT.	PACE	TIME	DIST.	INT.	PACE

WORKOUT LOG

NAME:
GOALS:
DATE:
STATS:
WEIGHT:

EXERCISE:	SETS	REPS	WEIGHT	REST	SETS	REPS	WEIGHT	REST	SETS	REPS	WEIGHT	REST	SETS	REPS	WEIGHT	REST

CARDIO:	TIME	DIST.	INT.	PACE	TIME	DIST.	INT.	PACE	TIME	DIST.	INT.	PACE	TIME	DIST.	INT.	PACE

WORKOUT LOG

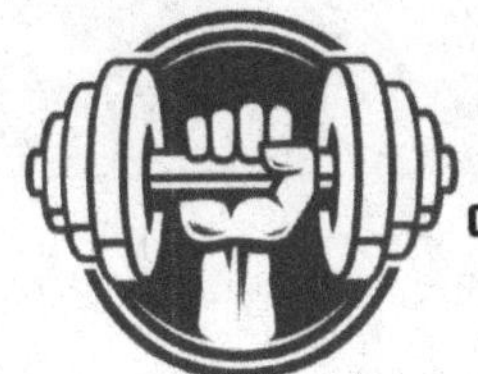

NAME:

GOALS:

DATE:

STATS:

WEIGHT:

EXERCISE:	SETS	REPS	WEIGHT	REST	SETS	REPS	WEIGHT	REST	SETS	REPS	WEIGHT	REST	SETS	REPS	WEIGHT	REST

CARDIO:	TIME	DIST.	INT.	PACE	TIME	DIST.	INT.	PACE	TIME	DIST.	INT.	PACE	TIME	DIST.	INT.	PACE

WORKOUT LOG

NAME:
GOALS:
DATE:
STATS:
WEIGHT:

EXERCISE:	SETS	REPS	WEIGHT	REST	SETS	REPS	WEIGHT	REST	SETS	REPS	WEIGHT	REST	SETS	REPS	WEIGHT	REST

CARDIO:	TIME	DIST.	INT.	PACE	TIME	DIST.	INT.	PACE	TIME	DIST.	INT.	PACE	TIME	DIST.	INT.	PACE

WORKOUT LOG

NAME:
GOALS:
DATE:
STATS:
WEIGHT:

EXERCISE:	SETS	REPS	WEIGHT	REST	SETS	REPS	WEIGHT	REST	SETS	REPS	WEIGHT	REST	SETS	REPS	WEIGHT	REST

CARDIO:	TIME	DIST.	INT.	PACE	TIME	DIST.	INT.	PACE	TIME	DIST.	INT.	PACE	TIME	DIST.	INT.	PACE

WORKOUT LOG

NAME:

GOALS:

DATE:

STATS:

WEIGHT:

EXERCISE:	SETS	REPS	WEIGHT	REST	SETS	REPS	WEIGHT	REST	SETS	REPS	WEIGHT	REST	SETS	REPS	WEIGHT	REST

CARDIO:	TIME	DIST.	INT.	PACE	TIME	DIST.	INT.	PACE	TIME	DIST.	INT.	PACE	TIME	DIST.	INT.	PACE

WORKOUT LOG

NAME: ___________________________

GOALS: __________________________

DATE: ____________________________

STATS: ___________________________

WEIGHT: __________________________

EXERCISE:	SETS	REPS	WEIGHT	REST	SETS	REPS	WEIGHT	REST	SETS	REPS	WEIGHT	REST	SETS	REPS	WEIGHT	REST

CARDIO:	TIME	DIST.	INT.	PACE	TIME	DIST.	INT.	PACE	TIME	DIST.	INT.	PACE	TIME	DIST.	INT.	PACE

WORKOUT LOG

NAME:
GOALS:
DATE:
STATS:
WEIGHT:

EXERCISE:	SETS	REPS	WEIGHT	REST	SETS	REPS	WEIGHT	REST	SETS	REPS	WEIGHT	REST	SETS	REPS	WEIGHT	REST

CARDIO:	TIME	DIST.	INT.	PACE	TIME	DIST.	INT.	PACE	TIME	DIST.	INT.	PACE	TIME	DIST.	INT.	PACE

WORKOUT LOG

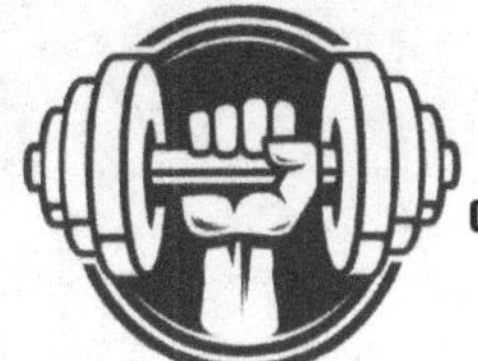

NAME:

GOALS:

DATE:

STATS:

WEIGHT:

EXERCISE:	SETS	REPS	WEIGHT	REST	SETS	REPS	WEIGHT	REST	SETS	REPS	WEIGHT	REST	SETS	REPS	WEIGHT	REST

CARDIO:	TIME	DIST.	INT.	PACE	TIME	DIST.	INT.	PACE	TIME	DIST.	INT.	PACE	TIME	DIST.	INT.	PACE

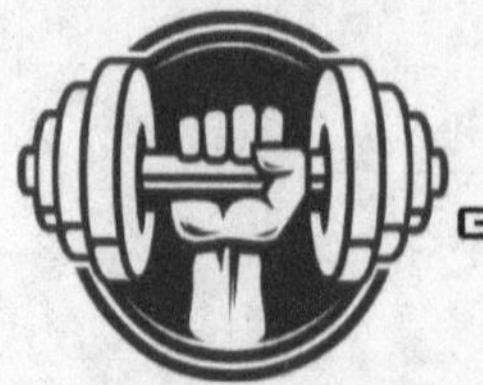

WORKOUT LOG

NAME: _______________________
GOALS: _______________________

DATE:
STATS:
WEIGHT:

EXERCISE:	SETS	REPS	WEIGHT	REST	SETS	REPS	WEIGHT	REST	SETS	REPS	WEIGHT	REST	SETS	REPS	WEIGHT	REST

CARDIO:	TIME	DIST.	INT.	PACE	TIME	DIST.	INT.	PACE	TIME	DIST.	INT.	PACE	TIME	DIST.	INT.	PACE

WORKOUT LOG

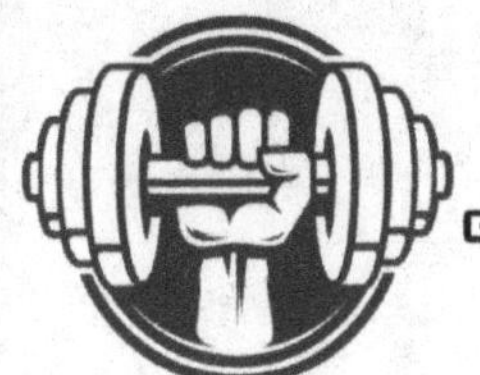

NAME:

GOALS:

DATE:

STATS:

WEIGHT:

EXERCISE:	SETS	REPS	WEIGHT	REST	SETS	REPS	WEIGHT	REST	SETS	REPS	WEIGHT	REST	SETS	REPS	WEIGHT	REST

CARDIO:	TIME	DIST.	INT.	PACE	TIME	DIST.	INT.	PACE	TIME	DIST.	INT.	PACE	TIME	DIST.	INT.	PACE

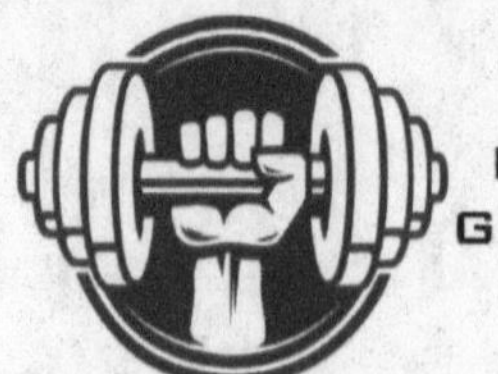

WORKOUT LOG

NAME:
GOALS:
DATE:
STATS:
WEIGHT:

EXERCISE:	SETS	REPS	WEIGHT	REST	SETS	REPS	WEIGHT	REST	SETS	REPS	WEIGHT	REST	SETS	REPS	WEIGHT	REST

CARDIO:	TIME	DIST.	INT.	PACE	TIME	DIST.	INT.	PACE	TIME	DIST.	INT.	PACE	TIME	DIST.	INT.	PACE

WORKOUT LOG

NAME:
GOALS:
DATE:
STATS:
WEIGHT:

EXERCISE:	SETS	REPS	WEIGHT	REST	SETS	REPS	WEIGHT	REST	SETS	REPS	WEIGHT	REST	SETS	REPS	WEIGHT	REST

CARDIO:	TIME	DIST.	INT.	PACE	TIME	DIST.	INT.	PACE	TIME	DIST.	INT.	PACE	TIME	DIST.	INT.	PACE

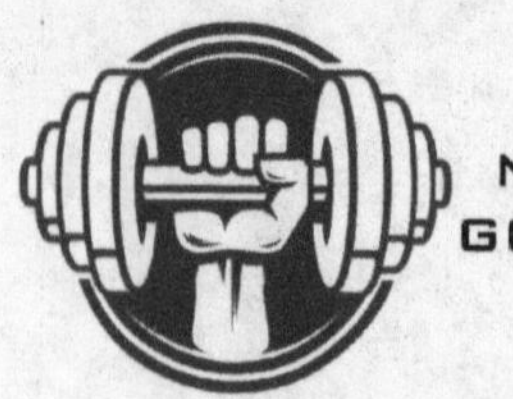

WORKOUT LOG

NAME: _______________________

GOALS: _______________________

DATE:

STATS:

WEIGHT:

EXERCISE:	SETS	REPS	WEIGHT	REST	SETS	REPS	WEIGHT	REST	SETS	REPS	WEIGHT	REST	SETS	REPS	WEIGHT	REST

CARDIO:	TIME	DIST.	INT.	PACE	TIME	DIST.	INT.	PACE	TIME	DIST.	INT.	PACE	TIME	DIST.	INT.	PACE

WORKOUT LOG

NAME:

GOALS:

DATE:

STATS:

WEIGHT:

EXERCISE:	SETS	REPS	WEIGHT	REST	SETS	REPS	WEIGHT	REST	SETS	REPS	WEIGHT	REST	SETS	REPS	WEIGHT	REST

CARDIO:	TIME	DIST.	INT.	PACE	TIME	DIST.	INT.	PACE	TIME	DIST.	INT.	PACE	TIME	DIST.	INT.	PACE

WORKOUT LOG

NAME:
GOALS:
DATE:
STATS:
WEIGHT:

EXERCISE:	SETS	REPS	WEIGHT	REST	SETS	REPS	WEIGHT	REST	SETS	REPS	WEIGHT	REST	SETS	REPS	WEIGHT	REST

CARDIO:	TIME	DIST.	INT.	PACE	TIME	DIST.	INT.	PACE	TIME	DIST.	INT.	PACE	TIME	DIST.	INT.	PACE

WORKOUT LOG

NAME:

GOALS:

DATE:

STATS:

WEIGHT:

EXERCISE:	SETS	REPS	WEIGHT	REST	SETS	REPS	WEIGHT	REST	SETS	REPS	WEIGHT	REST	SETS	REPS	WEIGHT	REST

CARDIO:	TIME	DIST.	INT.	PACE	TIME	DIST.	INT.	PACE	TIME	DIST.	INT.	PACE	TIME	DIST.	INT.	PACE

WORKOUT LOG

NAME:

GOALS:

DATE:

STATS:

WEIGHT:

EXERCISE:	SETS	REPS	WEIGHT	REST	SETS	REPS	WEIGHT	REST	SETS	REPS	WEIGHT	REST	SETS	REPS	WEIGHT	REST

CARDIO:	TIME	DIST.	INT.	PACE	TIME	DIST.	INT.	PACE	TIME	DIST.	INT.	PACE	TIME	DIST.	INT.	PACE

WORKOUT LOG

NAME:
GOALS:
DATE:
STATS:
WEIGHT:

EXERCISE:	SETS	REPS	WEIGHT	REST	SETS	REPS	WEIGHT	REST	SETS	REPS	WEIGHT	REST	SETS	REPS	WEIGHT	REST

CARDIO:	TIME	DIST.	INT.	PACE	TIME	DIST.	INT.	PACE	TIME	DIST.	INT.	PACE	TIME	DIST.	INT.	PACE

WORKOUT LOG

NAME:

GOALS:

DATE:

STATS:

WEIGHT:

EXERCISE:	SETS	REPS	WEIGHT	REST	SETS	REPS	WEIGHT	REST	SETS	REPS	WEIGHT	REST	SETS	REPS	WEIGHT	REST

CARDIO:	TIME	DIST.	INT.	PACE	TIME	DIST.	INT.	PACE	TIME	DIST.	INT.	PACE	TIME	DIST.	INT.	PACE

WORKOUT LOG

NAME:

GOALS:

DATE:

STATS:

WEIGHT:

EXERCISE:	SETS	REPS	WEIGHT	REST	SETS	REPS	WEIGHT	REST	SETS	REPS	WEIGHT	REST	SETS	REPS	WEIGHT	REST

CARDIO:	TIME	DIST.	INT.	PACE	TIME	DIST.	INT.	PACE	TIME	DIST.	INT.	PACE	TIME	DIST.	INT.	PACE

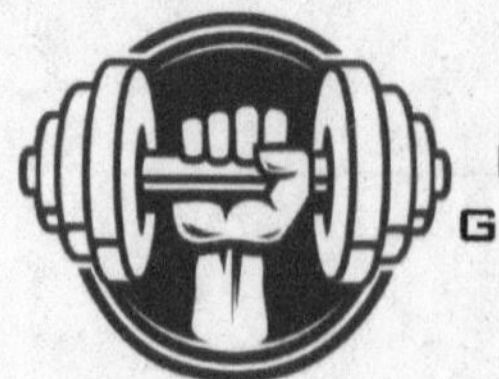

WORKOUT LOG

NAME:
GOALS:
DATE:
STATS:
WEIGHT:

EXERCISE:	SETS	REPS	WEIGHT	REST	SETS	REPS	WEIGHT	REST	SETS	REPS	WEIGHT	REST	SETS	REPS	WEIGHT	REST

CARDIO:	TIME	DIST.	INT.	PACE	TIME	DIST.	INT.	PACE	TIME	DIST.	INT.	PACE	TIME	DIST.	INT.	PACE

WORKOUT LOG

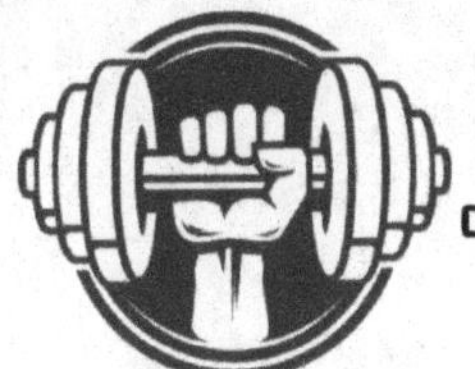

NAME:

GOALS:

DATE:

STATS:

WEIGHT:

EXERCISE:	SETS	REPS	WEIGHT	REST	SETS	REPS	WEIGHT	REST	SETS	REPS	WEIGHT	REST	SETS	REPS	WEIGHT	REST

CARDIO:	TIME	DIST.	INT.	PACE	TIME	DIST.	INT.	PACE	TIME	DIST.	INT.	PACE	TIME	DIST.	INT.	PACE

WORKOUT LOG

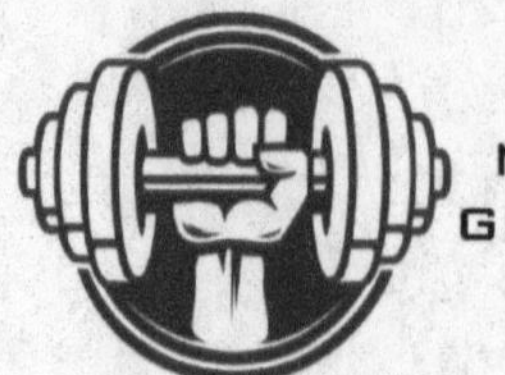

NAME:
GOALS:
DATE:
STATS:
WEIGHT:

EXERCISE:	SETS	REPS	WEIGHT	REST	SETS	REPS	WEIGHT	REST	SETS	REPS	WEIGHT	REST	SETS	REPS	WEIGHT	REST

CARDIO:	TIME	DIST.	INT.	PACE	TIME	DIST.	INT.	PACE	TIME	DIST.	INT.	PACE	TIME	DIST.	INT.	PACE

WORKOUT LOG

NAME:
GOALS:
DATE:
STATS:
WEIGHT:

EXERCISE:	SETS	REPS	WEIGHT	REST	SETS	REPS	WEIGHT	REST	SETS	REPS	WEIGHT	REST	SETS	REPS	WEIGHT	REST

CARDIO:	TIME	DIST.	INT.	PACE	TIME	DIST.	INT.	PACE	TIME	DIST.	INT.	PACE	TIME	DIST.	INT.	PACE

WORKOUT LOG

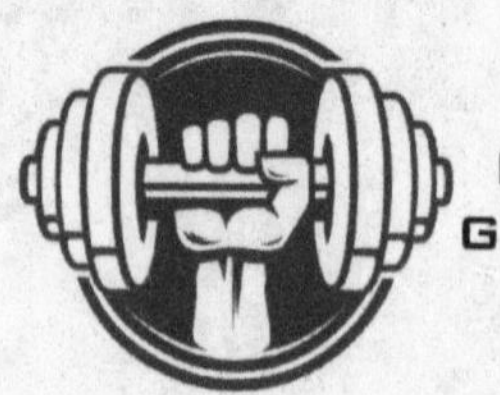

NAME:

GOALS:

DATE:

STATS:

WEIGHT:

EXERCISE:	SETS	REPS	WEIGHT	REST	SETS	REPS	WEIGHT	REST	SETS	REPS	WEIGHT	REST	SETS	REPS	WEIGHT	REST

CARDIO:	TIME	DIST.	INT.	PACE	TIME	DIST.	INT.	PACE	TIME	DIST.	INT.	PACE	TIME	DIST.	INT.	PACE

WORKOUT LOG

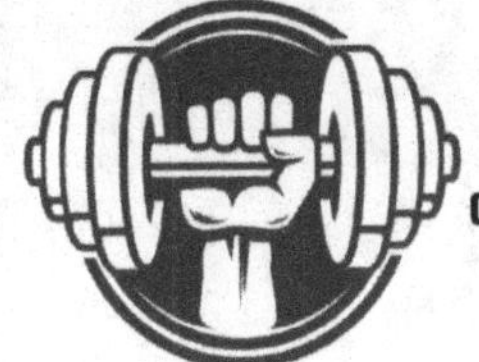

NAME:

GOALS:

DATE:

STATS:

WEIGHT:

EXERCISE:	SETS	REPS	WEIGHT	REST	SETS	REPS	WEIGHT	REST	SETS	REPS	WEIGHT	REST	SETS	REPS	WEIGHT	REST

CARDIO:	TIME	DIST.	INT.	PACE	TIME	DIST.	INT.	PACE	TIME	DIST.	INT.	PACE	TIME	DIST.	INT.	PACE

WORKOUT LOG

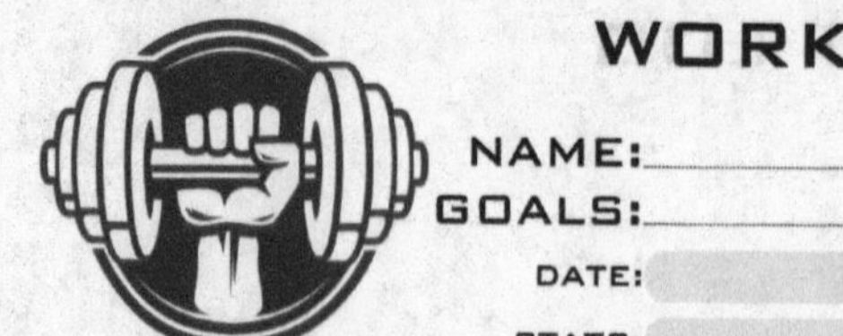

NAME:

GOALS:

DATE:

STATS:

WEIGHT:

EXERCISE:	SETS	REPS	WEIGHT	REST	SETS	REPS	WEIGHT	REST	SETS	REPS	WEIGHT	REST	SETS	REPS	WEIGHT	REST

CARDIO:	TIME	DIST.	INT.	PACE	TIME	DIST.	INT.	PACE	TIME	DIST.	INT.	PACE	TIME	DIST.	INT.	PACE

WORKOUT LOG

NAME:

GOALS:

DATE:

STATS:

WEIGHT:

EXERCISE:	SETS	REPS	WEIGHT	REST	SETS	REPS	WEIGHT	REST	SETS	REPS	WEIGHT	REST	SETS	REPS	WEIGHT	REST

CARDIO:	TIME	DIST.	INT.	PACE	TIME	DIST.	INT.	PACE	TIME	DIST.	INT.	PACE	TIME	DIST.	INT.	PACE

WORKOUT LOG

NAME:

GOALS:

DATE:

STATS:

WEIGHT:

EXERCISE:	SETS	REPS	WEIGHT	REST	SETS	REPS	WEIGHT	REST	SETS	REPS	WEIGHT	REST	SETS	REPS	WEIGHT	REST

CARDIO:	TIME	DIST.	INT.	PACE	TIME	DIST.	INT.	PACE	TIME	DIST.	INT.	PACE	TIME	DIST.	INT.	PACE